The Seafood and Dessert Cookbook For My Lean and Green Diet

50 delicious lean and green recipes for seafood and dessert to stay healthy and boost energy

Josephine Reed

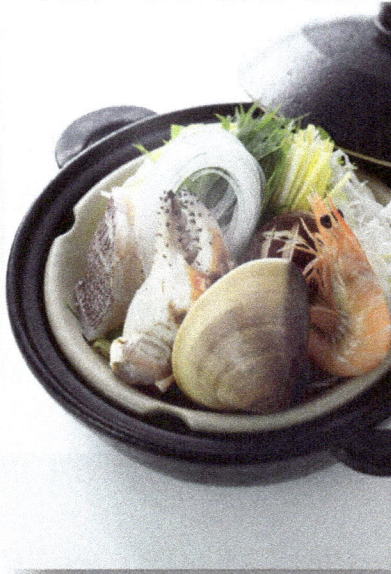

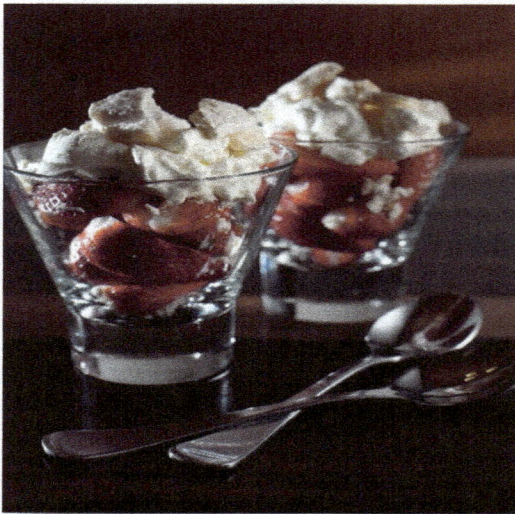

3

By reading this document, the reader agrees that under no circumstances is the author responsible for any losses, direct or indirect, which are incurred as a result of the use of information contained within this document, including, but not limited to, — errors, omissions, or inaccuracies.

Table of contents

5

Salmon & Veggie Salad

Prep Time: 15 minutes

Serve: 2

Ingredients:

- 6 ounces cooked wild salmon, chopped
- 1 cup cucumber, sliced
- 1 cup red bell-pepper, seeded and sliced ½ cup grape tomatoes, quartered
- 1 tablespoon scallion green, chopped
- 1 cup lettuce, torn
- 1 cup fresh spinach, torn
- 2 tablespoons olive oil
- 2 tablespoons fresh lemon juice
-

Instructions:

1.In a salad bowl, place all ingredients and gently toss to coat well.

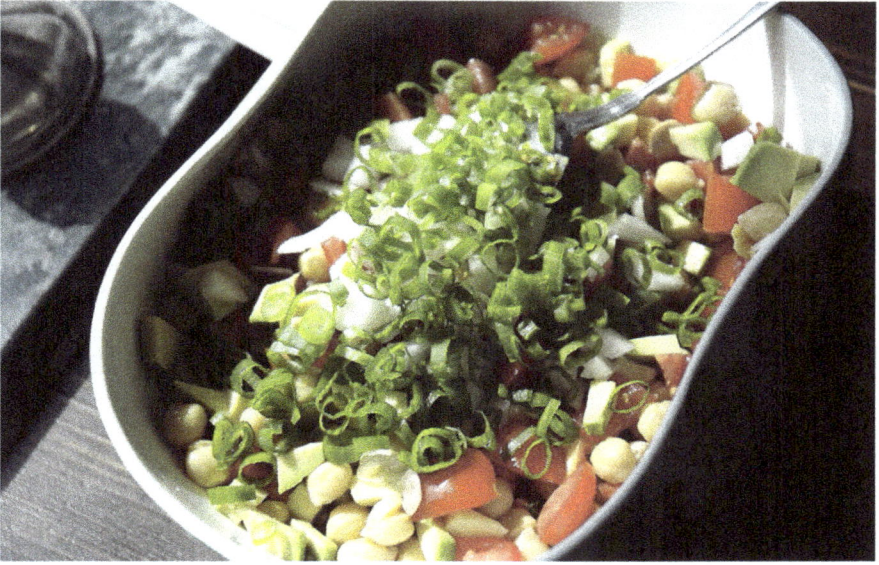

Tuna Salad

Prep Time: 15 minutes

Serve: 4

Ingredients:

For Dressing:

- 2 tablespoons fresh dill, minced
- 2 tablespoons olive oil
- 1 tablespoon fresh lime juice
- Salt and ground black pepper, to taste

For Salad:

- 4 cups fresh spinach, torn
- 2 (6-ounce) cans water-packed tuna, drained and flaked
- 6 hard-boiled eggs, peeled and sliced
- 1 cup tomato, chopped
- 1 large cucumber, sliced

Instructions:

1. For Dressing: place dill, oil, lime juice, salt, and black pepper in a small bowl and beat until well combined.

2.Divide the spinach onto serving plates and top each with tuna, egg, cucumber, and tomato.

3.Drizzle with dressing.

Shrimp & Greens Salad

Prep Time: 15 minutes

Cook Time: 6 minutes

Serve: 6

Ingredients:

- 3 tablespoons olive oil, divided
- 1 garlic clove, crushed and divided
- 2 tablespoons fresh rosemary, chopped
- 1-pound shrimp, peeled and deveined
- Salt and ground black pepper, as required
- 4 cups fresh arugula
- 2 cups lettuce, torn
- 2 tablespoons fresh lime juice

Instructions:

1.In a large wok, heat 1 normal spoon of oil over medium heat and sauté 1 garlic clove for about 1 minute.

2.Add the shrimp with salt and black pepper and cook for about 4-5 minutes.

3. Remove from the heat and place to cool aside.

4.Ina large bowl, add the shrimp, arugula, remaining oil, lime juice, salt and black pepper and gently, toss to coat.

Shrimp, Apple & Carrot Salad

Prep Time: 20 minutes

Cook Time: 3 minutes

Serve: 4

Ingredients:

- 12 medium shrimp
- 1½ cups Granny Smith apple, cored and sliced thinly 1½ cups carrot, peeled and cut into matchsticks
- ½ cup fresh mint leaves, chopped
- 2 tablespoons balsamic vinegar
- ¼ cup extra-virgin olive oil
- 1 teaspoon lemongrass, chopped
- 1 teaspoon garlic, minced
- 2 sprigs fresh cilantro, leaves separated and chopped

Instructions:

1.In a large pan of the salted boiling water, add the shrimp and lemon and cook for about 3 minutes.

2.Remove from the heat and drain the shrimp well.

3.Set aside to cool.

4.After cooling, peel and devein the shrimps.

5.Transfer the shrimp into a large bowl.

6.Add the remaining all ingredients except cilantro and gently, stir to combine.

7.Cover the bowl and refrigerate for about 1 hour.

8.Top with cilantro just before serving.

Shrimp & Green Beans Salad

Prep Time: 20 minutes

Cook Time: 8 minutes

Serve: 5

Ingredients:

For Shrimp:

- 2 tablespoons olive oil
- 2 tablespoons fresh key lime juice
- 4 large garlic cloves, peeled
- 2 sprigs fresh rosemary leaves
- ½ teaspoon garlic salt
- 20 large shrimp, peeled and deveined

For Salad:

- 1-pound fresh green beans, trimmed
- ¼ cup olive oil
- 1 onion, sliced
- Salt and ground black pepper, as required ½ cup garlic and herb feta cheese, crumbled

Instructions:

1.For shrimp marinade: in a blender, add all the ingredients except shrimp and pulse until smooth.

2.Transfer the marinade in a large bowl.

3.Add the shrimp and coat with marinade generously.

4. Cover the bowl and refrigerate for a minimum of 31 minutes to marinate.

5.Preheat the broiler of oven. Arrange the rack in top position of the oven. Line a large baking sheet with a piece of foil.

6.Place the shrimp with marinade onto the prepared baking sheet.

7.Broil for about 3-4 minutes per side.

8.Transfer the shrimp mixture into a bowl and refrigerate until using.

9.Meanwhile, For Salad: in a pan of the salted boiling water, add the green beans and cook for about 3-4 minutes.

10.Drain the green beans well and rinse under cold running water.

11.Transfer the green beans into a large bowl.

12.Add the onion, shrimp, salt and black pepper and stir to combine.

13.Cover and refrigerate to chill for about 1 hour.

14.Stir in cheese just before serving.

Shrimp & Olives Salad

Prep Time: 15 minutes

Cook Time: 3 minutes

Serve: 4

Ingredients:

- 1-pound shrimp, peeled and deveined
- 1 lemon, quartered
- 2 tablespoons olive oil
- 2 teaspoons fresh lemon juice
- Salt and freshly ground-black-pepper, to taste
- 2 tomatoe, sliced
- ¼ cup onion, sliced
- ¼ cup green olives
- ¼ cup fresh cilantro, chopped finely

Instructions:

1.In a tub of boiling water that is finely salted, add the quartered lemon.

2.Then, add the shrimp and cook for about 2-3 minutes or until pink and opaque.

3.With a slotted spoon, transfer the shrimp into a bowl of ice water to stop the cooking process.

4.Drain the shrimp completely and then pat dry with paper towels.

5.In a small bowl, add the oil, lemon juice, salt, and black pepper, and beat until well combined.

6.Divide the shrimp, tomato, onion, olives, and cilantro onto serving plates.

7.Drizzle with oil mixture.

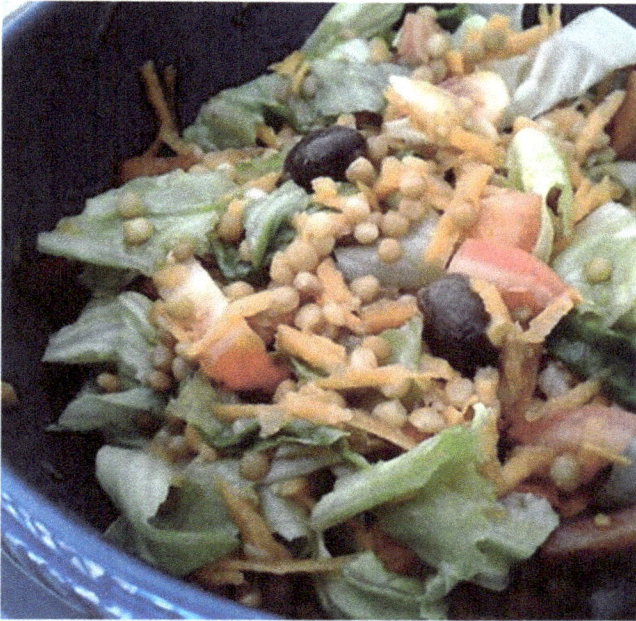

Shrimp & Arugula Salad

Prep Time: 15 minutes

Cook Time: 5 minutes

Serve: 4

Ingredients:

For Shrimp:

- 1-pound large shrimp, peeled and deveined ½ tablespoon fresh lemon juice

For Salad:

- 6 cups fresh arugula
- 2 tablespoons extra-virgin olive oil
- 1 tablespoons fresh lemon juice
- Salt and ground black pepper, as required

Instructions:

1.In a large pan of salted boiling water, add the shrimp and lemon juice and cook for about 2 minutes.

2. Withdraw the shrimp from the pan with a slotted-spoon and put it in an ice bath.

3.Drain the shrimp well.

4.In a large bowl, add the shrimp, arugula, oil, lemon juice, salt and black pepper and gently, toss to coat.

Shrimp & Veggies Salad

Prep Time: 20 minutes

Cook Time: 5 minutes

Serve: 6

Ingredients:

For Dressing:

- 2 tablespoons natural almond butter
- 1 garlic clove, crushed
- 1 tablespoon fresh cilantro, chopped
- 2 tablespoons fresh lime juice
- 1 tablespoon maple syrup
- ½ teaspoon cayenne pepper
- ¼ teaspoon salt
- 1 tablespoon water
- 1/3 cup olive oil

For Salad:

- 1-pound shrimp, peeled and deveined Salt and ground black pepper, as required
- 1 teaspoon olive oil
- 1 cup carrot, peeled and julienned

- 1 cup red cabbage, shredded
- 1 cup green cabbage, shredded
- 1 cup cucumber, julienned
- 4 cups fresh baby arugula
- ¼ cup fresh basil, chopped
- ¼ cup fresh cilantro, chopped
- 4 cups lettuce, torn
- ¼ cup almonds, chopped

Instructions:

1.For Dressing: in a bowl, add all ingredients except oil and beat until well combined.

2.Slowly, add oil, beating continuously until smooth.

3.For Salad: in a bowl, add shrimp, salt, black pepper and oil and toss to coat well.

4. Heat a skillet over medium-high heat and cook the shrimp on each side for about two minutes.

5.Detach from the heat to cool and set aside.

6.In a large serving bowl, add all the cooked shrimp, remaining salad ingredients and dressing and toss to coat well.

Salmon Lettuce Wraps

Prep Time: 10 minutes

Serve: 2

Ingredients:

- ¼ cup low-fat mozzarella cheese, cubed ¼ cup tomato, chopped
- 2 tablespoons fresh dill, chopped
- 1 teaspoon fresh lemon juice
- Salt, as required
- 4 lettuce leaves
- 1/3 pound cooked salmon, chopped

Instructions:

1.In a small bowl, combine mozzarella, tomato, dill, lemon juice, and salt until well combined.

2.Arrange the lettuce leaves onto serving plates.

3.Divide the salmon and tomato mixture over each lettuce leaf and serve immediately.

Tuna Burgers

Prep Time: 15 minutes

Cook Time: 6 minutes

Serve: 2

Ingredients:

- 1 (15-ounce) can water-packed tuna, drained
- ½ celery stalk, chopped
- 2 tablespoon fresh parsley, chopped
- 1 teaspoon fresh dill, chopped
- 2 tablespoon walnuts, chopped
- 2 tablespoon mayonnaise
- 1 egg, beaten
- 1 tablespoon butter
- 3 cups lettuce

Instructions:

1.For Burgers: add all ingredients except the butter and lettuce in a bowl and mix until well combined.

2.Make 2 equal-sized patties from mixture.

3.In a frying pan, melt butter over medium heat and cook the patties for about 2-3 minutes.

4.Carefully flip the side and cook for about 2-3 minutes.

5.Divide the lettuce onto serving plates.

6.Top each plate with 1 burger and serve.

Spicy Salmon

Prep Time: 105 minutes

Cook Time: 8 minutes

Serve: 4

Ingredients:

- 4 tablespoons extra-virgin olive oil, divided
- 2 tablespoons fresh lemon juice
- 1 teaspoon ground turmeric
- 1 teaspoon ground cumin
- Salt and ground black pepper, as required
- 4 (4-ounce) boneless, skinless salmon fillets
- 6 cups fresh arugula

Instructions:

1.In a bowl, mix together 2 normal spoons of oil, lemon juice, turmeric, cumin, salt and black pepper.

2.Add the salmon fillets and coat with the oil mixture generously. Set aside.

3.In a non-stick wok, heat remaining oil over medium heat.

4.Place salmon fillets, skin-side down and cook for about 3-5 minutes.

5.Change the side and cook for about 2-3 minutes more.

6.Divide the salmon onto serving plates and serve immediately alongside the arugula.

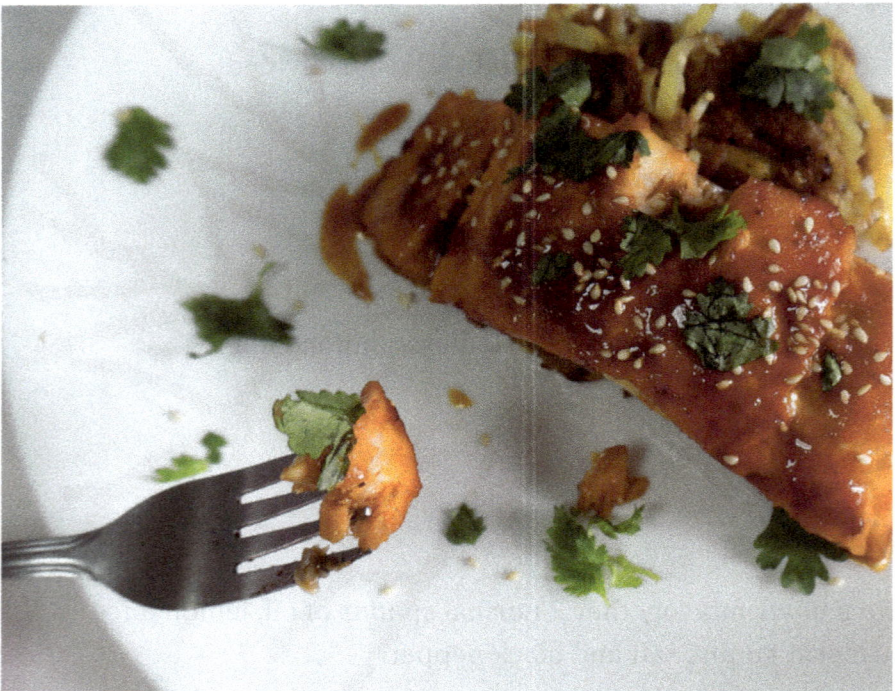

Lemony Salmon

Prep Time: 10 minutes

Cook Time: 14 minutes

Serve: 4

Ingredients:

- 2 garlic cloves, minced
- 1 tablespoon fresh lemon zest, grated
- 2 tablespoons olive oil
- 2 tablespoons fresh lemon juice
- Salt and ground black pepper, to taste
- 4 (6-ounce) boneless, skinless salmon fillets
- 6 cups fresh spinach

Instructions:

1. Preheat the grill to medium-high heat.

2. Grease the grill grate.

3. In a bowl, place all-ingredients except for salmon and spinach and mix well.

4.Add the salmon fillets and coat with garlic mixture generously.

5.Grill the salmon fillets for about 6-7 minutes per side.

6.Serve immediately alongside the spinach.

Zesty Salmon

Prep Time: 10 minutes

Cook Time: 10 minutes

Serve: 4

Ingredients:

- 1 tablespoon butter, melted
- 1 tablespoon fresh lemon juice
- 1 teaspoon Worcestershire sauce
- 1 teaspoon lemon zest, grated finely.
- 4 (6-ounce) salmon fillets
- Salt and ground black pepper, to taste

Instructions:

1.In a baking dish, place butter, lemon juice, Worcestershire sauce, and lemon zest, and mix well.

2.Coat the fillets with mixture and then arrange skin side-up in the baking dish.

3.Set aside for about 15 minutes.

4.Preheat the broiler of oven.

5.Arrange the oven rack about 6-inch from heating element.

6.Line a broiler pan with a piece of foil.

7.Remove the salmon fillets from baking dish and season with salt and black pepper.

8.Arrange the salmon fillets onto the prepared broiler pan, skin side down.

9.Broil for about 8-10 minutes.

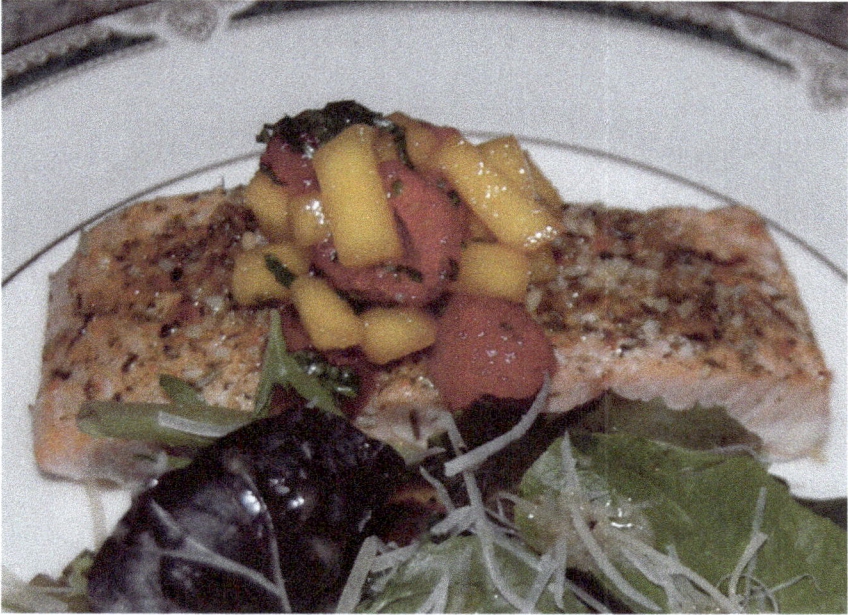

Stuffed Salmon

Prep Time: 15 minutes

Cook Time: 16 minutes

Serve: 4

Ingredients:

For Salmon:

- 4 (6-ounce) skinless salmon fillets
- Salt and ground black pepper, as required
- 2 tablespoons fresh lemon juice
- 2 tablespoons olive oil, divided
- 1 tablespoon unsalted butter

For Filling:

- 4 ounces low-fat cream cheese, softened
- ¼ cup low-fat Parmesan cheese, grated finely
- 4 ounces frozen spinach, thawed and squeezed
- 2 teaspoons garlic, minced
- Salt and ground black pepper, as required

Instructions:

1.Season each salmon-fillet with salt and black-pepper and then, drizzle with lemon juice and 1 tablespoon of oil.

2.Arrange the salmon fillets onto a smooth surface.

3.With a sharp knife, cut a pocket into each salmon fillet about ¾ of the way through, take care not to cut the whole way.

4.For filling: in a bowl, add the cream cheese, Parmesan cheese, spinach, garlic, salt and black pepper and mix well.

5.Place about 1-2 tablespoons of spinach mixture into each salmon pocket and spread evenly.

6.In a skillet, heat the remaining oil and butter over medium-high heat and cook the salmon fillets for about 6-8 minutes per side.

7.Remove the salmon fillets from heat and transfer onto the serving plates.

Salmon with Asparagus

Prep Time: 10 minutes

Cook Time: 20 minutes

Serve: 6

Ingredients:

- 6 (4-ounce) salmon fillets
- 2 tablespoons extra-virgin olive oil
- 3 tablespoons fresh parsley, minced
- ¼ teaspoon ginger powder
- Salt and freshly ground black-pepper, to taste
- 1½ pounds fresh asparagus

Instructions:

1.Preheat your oven to 400 degrees.

2.Grease a large baking dish.

3.In a bowl, place all-ingredients and mix well.

4.Arrange the salmon fillets into prepared baking dish in a single layer.

5.Bake for approximately 16-21 minutes or until desired doneness of salmon.

6.Meanwhile, in a pan of the boiling water, add asparagus and cook for about 4-5 minutes.

7.Drain the asparagus well.

8.Divide the asparagus onto serving plates evenly and top each with 1 salmon fillet and serve.

Salmon Parcel

Prep Time: 15 minutes

Cook Time: 20 minutes

Serve: 6

Ingredients:

- 6 (4-ounce) salmon-fillets
- Salt and freshly ground-black-pepper, to taste 1 yellow bell pepper, seeded and cubed
- 1 red bell pepper, seeded and cubed
- 4 plum tomatoes, cubed
- 1 small onion, sliced thinly
- ½ cup fresh parsley, chopped
- ¼ cup extra-virgin olive oil
- 2 tablespoons fresh lemon juice

Instructions:

1.Preheat your oven to 400 degrees F.

2.Arrange 6 pieces of foil onto a smooth surface.

3.Place one salmon-fillet on each piece of foil and sprinkle with salt and black pepper.

4.In a bowl, mix together bell peppers, tomato and onion.

5.Place veggie mixture over each fillet evenly and top with parsley and capers evenly.

6.Drizzle with oil and lemon juice.

7.Fold the each piece of foil around salmon mixture to seal it.

8.Arrange the foil packets onto a large baking sheet in a single layer.

9.Bake for approximately 25 minutes.

10.Remove from the oven and place the foil packets onto serving plates.

11.Carefully unwrap each foil packet and serve.

Salmon with Cauliflower Mash

Prep Time: 15 minutes

Cook Time: 20 minutes

Serve: 4

Ingredients:

For Cauliflower Mash:

- 1-pound cauliflower, cut into florets
- 1 tablespoon extra-virgin olive oil
- 3 garlic cloves, minced
- 1 teaspoon fresh thyme leaves
- Salt and freshly ground black-pepper, to taste

For Salmon:

- 1 (1-inch) piece fresh ginger, grated finely
- 1 tablespoon honey
- 1 tablespoon fresh lemon juice
- 1 tablespoon Dijon mustard
- 2 tablespoons olive oil
- 4 (6-ounce) salmon fillets
- 2 tablespoons fresh parsley, chopped

Instructions:

1.For mash: in a large saucepan of water, arrange a steamer basket and bring to a boil.

2.Place the cauliflower florets in steamer basket and steam covered for about 10 minutes.

3.Drain the cauliflower and set aside.

4.In a small-frying pan, heat the oil over-medium heat and sauté the garlic for about 2 minutes.

5.Remove the frying pan from heat and transfer the garlic oil in a large food processor.

6.Add the cauliflower, thyme, salt and black-pepper and pulse until smooth.

7.Transfer the cauliflower mash into a bowl and set aside.

8.Meanwhile, in a bowl, mix together ginger, honey, lemon juice and Dijon mustard. Set aside.

9.In a large non-stick skillet, heat olive-oil over medium-high heat and cook the salmon fillets for about 3-4 minutes per side.

10.Stir in honey mixture and immediately remove from heat.

11.Divide warm cauliflower mash onto serving plates.

12. Top each plate with one salmon fillet and serve.

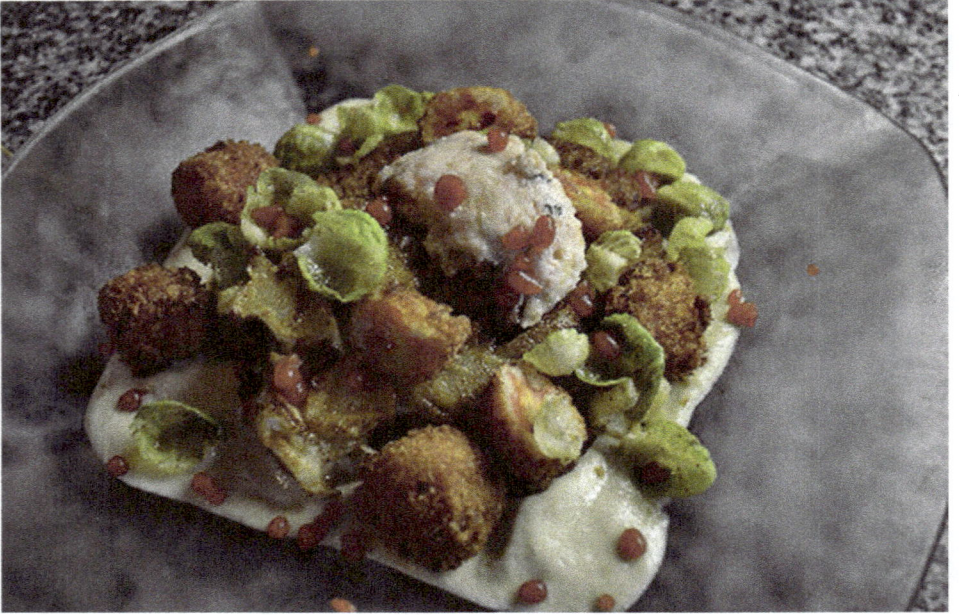

Salmon with Salsa

Prep Time: 15 minutes

Cook Time: 8 minutes

Serve: 4

Ingredients:

For Salsa:

- 2 large ripe avocados, peeled, pitted and cut into small chunks
- 1 small tomato, chopped
- 2 tablespoons red onion, chopped finely ¼ cup fresh cilantro, chopped finely
- 1 tablespoon jalapeño pepper, seeded and minced finely
- 1 garlic clove, minced finely
- 3 tablespoon fresh lime juice
- Salt and ground black pepper, as required

For Salmon:

- 4 (5-ounce) (1-inch thick) salmon fillets
- Sea salt and ground black-pepper, as required
- 3 tablespoons olive oil
- 1 tablespoon fresh rosemary leaves, chopped

- 1 tablespoon fresh lemon juice

Instructions:

1.For salsa: add all ingredients in a bowl and gently, stir to combine.

2.With a plastic-wrap, cover the bowl and refrigerate before serving.

3.For salmon: season each salmon fillet with salt and black pepper generously.

4.In a big-skillet, heat the oil over medium-high heat.

5.Place the salmon fillets, skins side up and cook for about 4 minutes.

6.Carefully change the side of each salmon fillet and cook for about 4 minutes more.

7.Stir in the rosemary and lemon juice and remove from the heat.

8.Divide the salsa onto serving plates evenly.

9.To each plate with 1 salmon fillet and serve.

Walnut Crusted Salmon

Prep Time: 15 minutes

Cook Time: 20 minutes

Serve: 2

Ingredients:

- ½ cup walnuts
- 1 tablespoon fresh dill, chopped
- 2 tablespoons fresh lemon rind, grated
- Salt and ground black pepper, as required
- 1 tablespoon coconut oil, melted
- 3-4 tablespoons Dijon mustard
- 4 (3-ounce) salmon fillets
- 4 teaspoons fresh lemon juice
- 3 cups fresh baby spinach

Instructions:

1.Preheat your oven to 350 degrees F.

2.Line the parchment paper with a large baking sheet.

3.Place the walnuts in a food processor and pulse until chopped roughly.

4.Add the dill, lemon rind, garlic salt, black pepper, and butter, and pulse until a crumbly mixture forms.

5.Place the salmon fillets onto prepared baking sheet in a single layer, skin-side down.

6.Coat the top of each salmon-fillet with Dijon mustard.

7.Place the walnut mixture over each fillet and gently, press into the surface of salmon.

8.Bake for approximately 15–20 minutes.

9.Remove the salmon fillets from oven and transfer onto the serving plates.

10. Drizzle with the lemon juice and serve alongside the spinach.

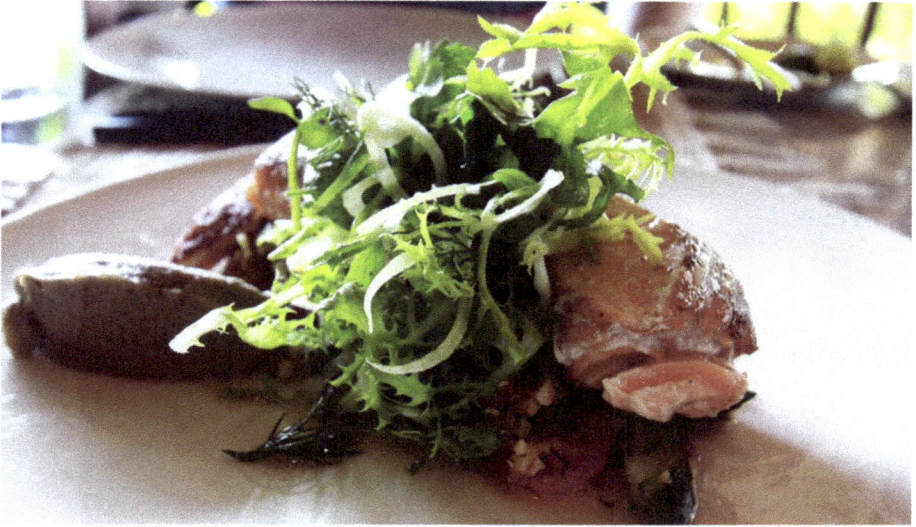

Garlicky Tilapia

Prep Time: 10 minutes

Cook Time: 5 minutes

Serve: 4

Ingredients:

- 2 tablespoons olive oil
- 4 (5-ounce) tilapia fillets
- 3 garlic cloves, minced
- 1 tablespoon fresh ginger, minced
- 2-3 tablespoons low-sodium chicken broth Salt and ground black pepper, to taste
- 6 cups fresh baby spinach

Instructions:

1.In a big sauté-pan, heat the oil over medium heat and cook the tilapia fillets for about 3 minutes.

2.Flip the side and stir in the garlic and ginger.

3.Cook for about 1-2 minutes.

4.Add the broth and cook for about 2-3 more minutes.

5.Stir in salt and black pepper and remove from heat.

6.Serve hot alongside the spinach.

Tilapia Piccata

Prep Time: 15 minutes

Cook Time: 8 minutes

Serve: 4

Ingredients:

- 3 tablespoons fresh lemon juice
- 2 tablespoons olive oil
- 2 garlic cloves, minced
- ½ teaspoon lemon zest, grated
- 2 teaspoons capers, drained
- 2 tablespoons fresh basil, minced
- 4 (6-ounce) tilapia fillets
- Salt and ground black pepper, as required 6 cups fresh baby kale

Instructions:

1.Preheat the broiler of the oven.

2.Arrange an oven rack about 4-inch from the heating element.

3.Grease a broiler pan.

4.In a little-bowl, add the lemon juice, oil, garlic and lemon zest and beat until well combined.

5.Add the capers and basil and stir to combine.

6.Reserve 2 tablespoons of mixture in a small bowl.

7.Coat the fish fillets with remaining capers mixture and sprinkle with salt and black pepper.

8.Place the tilapia fillets onto the broiler pan and broil for about 3-4 minutes side.

9.Remove from the oven and place the fish fillets onto serving plates.

10. Drizzle with reserved capers mixture and serve alongside the kale.

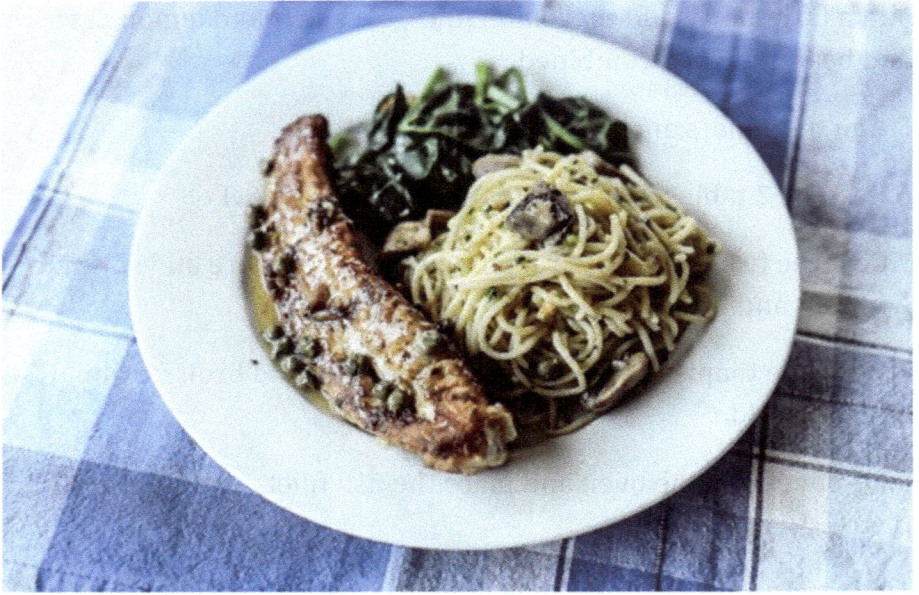

Cod in Dill Sauce

Prep Time: 10 minutes

Cook Time: 13 minutes

Serve: 2

Ingredients:

- 2 (6-ounce) cod fillets
- 1 teaspoon onion powder
- Salt and ground black pepper, as required 3 tablespoons butter, divided
- 2 garlic cloves, minced
- 1-2 lemon slices
- 2 teaspoons fresh dill weed
- 3 cups fresh spinach, torn

Instructions:

1. Season each cod fillet evenly with the onion powder, salt and black pepper.

2. In a medium skillet, heat 1 normal spoon of oil over high heat and cook the cod fillets for about 4-5 minutes per side.

3. Transfer the cod fillets onto a plate.

4.Meanwhile, in a frying-pan, heat the remaining oil over low heat and sauté the garlic and lemon slices for about 40-60 seconds.

5.Stir in the cooked cod fillets and dill and cook, covered for about 1-2 minutes.

6.Remove the cod fillets from heat and transfer onto the serving plates.

7.Top with the pan sauce and serve immediately alongside the spinach.

Cod & Veggies Bake

Prep Time: 15 minutes

Cook Time: 20 minutes

Serve: 4

Ingredients:

- 1 teaspoon olive oil
- ½ cup onion, minced
- 1 cup zucchini, chopped
- 1 garlic clove, minced
- 2 tablespoons fresh basil, chopped
- 2 cups fresh tomatoes, chopped
- Salt and ground black pepper, as required
- 4 (6-ounce) cod steaks
- 1/3 cup feta cheese, crumbled

Instructions:

1.Preheat your oven to 450 degrees F.

2.Grease a large shallow baking dish.

3.In a skillet, heat oil over-medium heat and sauté the onion, zucchini and garlic for about 4-5 minutes.

4.Stir in the basil, tomatoes, salt and black pepper and immediately remove from heat.

5.Place the cod steaks into prepared baking dish in a single layer and top with tomato mixture evenly.

6.Sprinkle with the cheese evenly.

7.Bake for approximately 16 minutes or until desired doneness.

Cod & Veggie Pizza

Prep Time: 20 minutes

Cook Time: 1 hour

Serve: 3

Ingredients:

For Base:

- Olive oil cooking spray
- ¼ cup oat flour
- 2 teaspoons dried rosemary, crushed
- Freshly ground black pepper, to taste
- 4 egg whites
- 2½ teaspoons olive oil
- ½ cup low-fat Parmesan cheese, grated freshly 2 cups zucchini, grated and squeezed

For Topping:

- 1 cup tomato paste
- 1 teaspoon fresh rosemary, minced
- 1 teaspoon fresh basil, minced
- Freshly ground black pepper, to taste
- 4 cups fresh mushrooms, chopped
- 1 tomato, chopped

- 3 ounces boneless cod fillet, chopped
- 1½ cups onion, sliced into rings
- 1 red bell pepper, seeded and chopped
- 1 green bell-pepper, seeded and chopped 1/3 cup low-fat mozzarella, shredded

Instructions:

1.Preheat your oven to 400 degrees F.

2.Grease a pie dish with cooking spray.

3.For base: in a large bowl, add all the ingredients and mix until well combined.

4.Transfer the mixture into prepared pie dish and press to smooth the surface.

5.Bake for approximately 40 minutes.

6. Remove from the oven to cool and set aside for at least 15 minutes.

7.Carefully turn out the crust onto a baking sheet.

8.For topping: in s bowl, add tomato paste, herbs and black pepper.

9.Spread tomato sauce mixture over crust evenly.

10.Arrange the vegetables over tomato sauce, followed by the cheese.

11.Bake for about 21 minutes or until cheese is melted.

Garlicky Haddock

Prep Time: 10 minutes

Cook Time: 11 minutes

Serve: 2

Ingredients:

- 2 tablespoons olive oil, divided
- 4 garlic cloves, minced and divided
- 1 teaspoon fresh ginger, grated finely
- 2 (4-ounce) haddock fillets
- Salt and freshly ground black-pepper, to taste 3 C. fresh baby spinach

Instructions:

1.In a skillet, heat one normal spoon of oil over medium heat and sauté 2 garlic cloves and ginger for about 1 minute.

2.Add the haddock fillets, salt and black pepper and cook for about 3-5 minutes per side or until desired doneness.

3. Meanwhile, heat the remaining oil over medium heat in another skillet, and heat and sauté the remaining garlic for about 1 minute.

4.Ad the spinach, salt and black pepper and cook for about 4-5 minutes.

5.Divide the spinach onto serving plates and top each with 1 haddock fillet.

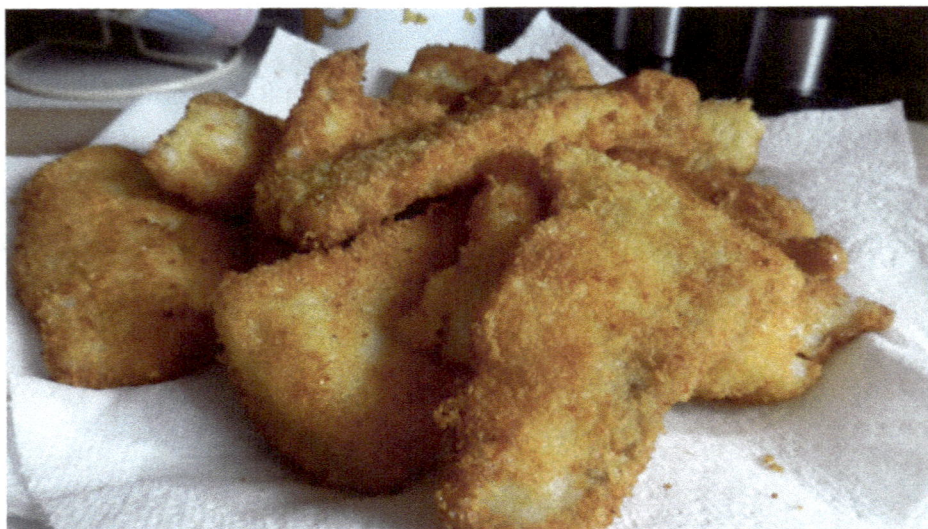

DESSERT

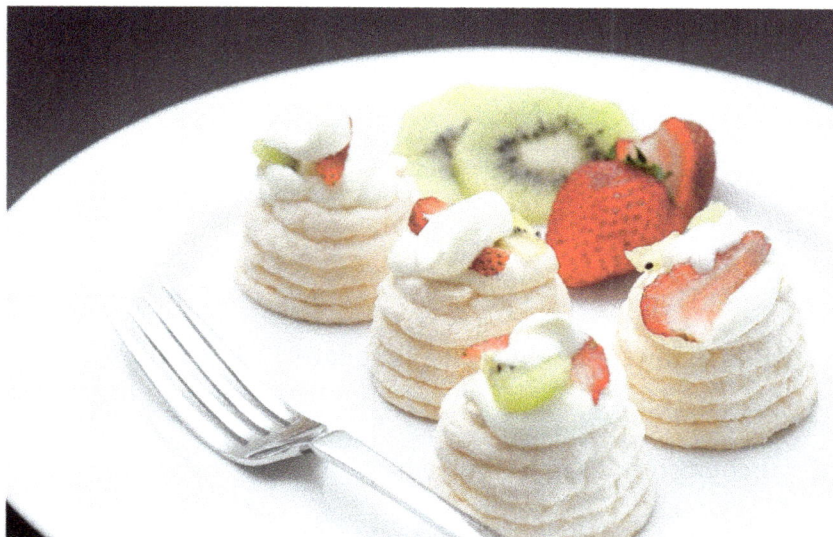

Sweet Potato Muffins Fueling Hack

Prep Time: 15 minutes

Cook Time: 15 minutes

Serve: 4

Ingredients:

- 1 packet Honey Sweet potatoes
- 2 Tablespoon liquid egg (like Eggbeaters) 1/2 C water
- 1/4 tsp baking powder
- 2 pinches Sinful Cinnamon Seasoning

Instructions:

1.Preheat oven to 400 degrees.

2.Sift the baking powder into the liquid egg.

3.Puree the sweet potatoes and add to the egg/baking powder mix.

4.Go on a light run and bring the water to a boil; add to the potato mix.

5.Bring in the cinnamon and the seasoning.

6.Whisk until well-combined.

7.Fill about ¾ of the way with the muffin cups with this mix.

8.Place into the oven for 15 minutes.

Nutrition: Energy (calories): 189 kcal Protein: 39.52 g Fat: 10.02 g
Carbohydrates: 1.98 g Calcium, Ca44 mg Magnesium, Mg48 mg
Phosphorus, P200 mg

Decadently Dark Chocolate Mousse

Prep Time: 10 minutes

Cook Time: 0 minutes

Serve: 2

Ingredients:

- 2 ripe avocados
- One-half cup unsweetened, dark cocoa powder 1 T vanilla
- One-fourth cup stevia powder
- One-fourth cup Unsweetened pinch of almond milk salt

Instructions:

1.Combine all ingredients into a high-speed blender and blend until smooth. (This can be done in a food processor as well. I would skip the blending and just mash the ingredients with a mortar and pestle.)

2.Preserve this mousse in a closed container in the fridge for up to 5 days.

Nutrition: Energy (calories): 466 kcal Protein: 9.27 g Fat: 38.35 g Carbohydrates: 31.21 g Calcium, Ca132 mg Magnesium, Mg154 mg Phosphorus, P259 mg

Chocolate Bars

Prep Time: 10 minutes

Cook Time: 20 minutes

Serve: 16

Ingredients:

- 15 oz cream cheese, softened
- 15 oz unsweetened dark chocolate
- 1 tsp vanilla
- 10 drops liquid stevia

Instructions:

1.Grease 8-inch square dish and set aside.

2.In a saucepan, dissolve chocolate over low heat.

3.Add stevia and vanilla and stir well.

4.Remove pan from heat and set aside.

5.Add cream cheese into the blender and blend until smooth.

6.Add melted chocolate mixture into the cream cheese and blend until just combined.

7.Transfer mixture into the prepared dish and spread evenly, and place in the refrigerator until firm.

Nutrition: Calories: 230 Fat: 24 g Carbs: 7.5 g Sugar: 0.1 g Protein: 6 g Cholesterol: 29 mg

Blueberry Muffins

Prep Time: 15 minutes

Cook Time: 35 minutes

Serve: 12

Ingredients:

- 2 eggs
- 1/2 cup fresh blueberries
- 1 cup heavy cream
- 2 cups almond flour
- 1/4 tsp lemon zest
- 1/2 tsp lemon extract
- 1 tsp baking powder
- 5 drops stevia
- 1/4 cup butter, melted

Instructions:

1. heat the cooker to 350 F. Line muffin tin with cupcake liners and set aside.

2. Add eggs into the bowl and whisk until mix.

3. Add remaining ingredients and mix to combine.

4.Pour mixture into the prepared muffin tin and bake for 25 minutes.

Nutrition: Calories: 190 Fat: 17 g Carbs: 5 g Sugar: 1 g Protein: 5 g Cholesterol: 55 mg

Chia Pudding

Prep Time: 20 minutes

Cook Time: 0 minutes

Serve: 2

Ingredients:

- 4 tbsp chia seeds
- 1 cup unsweetened coconut milk
- 1/2 cup raspberries

Instructions:

1.Add raspberry and coconut milk into a blender and blend until smooth.

2.Pour mixture into the glass jar.

3.Add chia seeds in a jar and stir well.

4.Seal the jar with a lid and shake well and place in the refrigerator for 3 hours.

5.Serve chilled and enjoy.

Nutrition: Calories: 360 Fat: 33 g Carbs: 13 g Sugar: 5 g Protein: 6 g Cholesterol: 0 mg

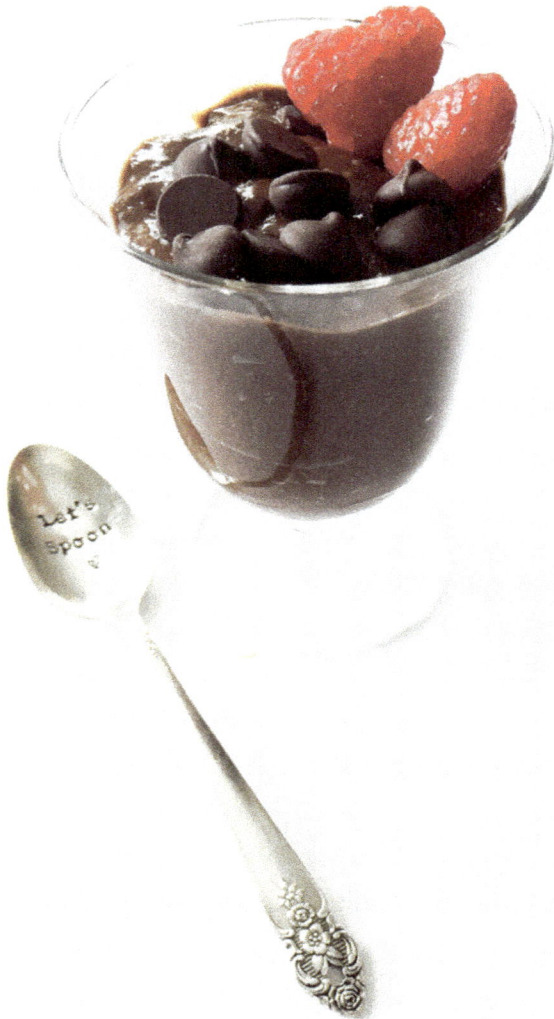

Avocado Pudding

Prep Time: 20 minutes

Cook Time: 0 minutes

Serve: 8

Ingredients:

- 2 ripe avocados, pitted and cut into pieces
- 1 tbsp fresh lime juice
- 14 oz can coconut milk
- 2 tsp liquid stevia
- 2 tsp vanilla

Instructions:

1.Inside the blender, Add all ingredients and blend until smooth.

Nutrition: Calories: 317 Fat: 30 g Carbs: 9 g Sugar: 0.5 g Protein: 3 g Cholesterol: 0 mg

Delicious Brownie Bites

Prep Time: 20 minutes

Cook Time: 0 minutes

Serve: 13

Ingredients:

- 1/4 cup unsweetened chocolate chips
- 1/4 cup unsweetened cocoa powder
- 1 cup pecans, chopped
- 1/2 cup almond butter
- 1/2 tsp vanilla
- 1/4 cup monk fruit sweetener
- 1/8 tsp pink salt

Instructions:

1.Add pecans, sweetener, vanilla, almond butter, cocoa powder, and salt into the food processor and process until well combined.

2.Transfer the brownie mixture into the large bowl. Add chocolate chips and fold well.

3.Make small round shape balls from brownie mixture and place them onto a baking tray.

4.Place in the freezer for 20 minutes.

Nutrition: Calories: 108 Fat: 9 g Carbs: 4 g Sugar: 1 g Protein: 2 g Cholesterol: 0 mg

Fresh Strawberry Salad Dressing

Prep Time: 10 minutes

Cook Time: 0 minutes

Serve: 2

Ingredients:

- 1 C – Fresh Ripe Strawberries
- 1 T – Balsamic Vinegar Mosto Cotto 2 T – Lemon Oil
- 1/4 tsp Peppercorns 1 Pinch Sea Salt

Instructions:

1.Put all the ingredients into a food-processor or blender and blend until creamy, then transfer to a serving bowl or pitcher for serving.

Nutrition: Energy (calories): 339 kcal Protein: 0.57 g Fat: 1.83 g Carbohydrates: 82.37 g Calcium, Ca12 mg Magnesium, Mg13 mg Phosphorus, P21 mg

Pumpkin_Balls

Prep Time: 15 minutes

Cook Time: 0 minutes

Serve: 18

Ingredients:

- 1 cup almond butter
- 5 drops liquid stevia
- 2 tbsp coconut flour
- 2 tbsp pumpkin puree
- 1 tsp pumpkin pie spice

Instructions:

1. Mix pumpkin puree in a large bowl and almond butter until well combined.

2. Add liquid stevia, pumpkin pie spice, and coconut flour and mix well.

3. Make little balls from the mixture and place them on a baking tray.

4. Place in the freezer for 1 hour.

Nutrition: Calories: 96 Fat: 8 g Carbs: 4 g Sugar: 1 g Protein: 2 g Cholesterol: 0 mg

Smooth Peanut Butter Cream

Prep Time: 10 minutes

Cook Time: 0 minutes

Serve: 8

Ingredients:

- 1/4 cup peanut butter
- 4 overripe bananas, chopped
- 1/3 cup cocoa powder
- 1/4 tsp vanilla extract
- 1/8 tsp salt

Instructions:

1. In the blender, add all the listed ingredients and blend until smooth.

Nutrition: Calories: 101 Fat: 5 g Carbs: 14 g Sugar: 7 g Protein: 3 g Cholesterol: 0 mg

Vanilla Avocado Popsicles

Prep Time: 20 minutes

Cook Time: 0 minutes

Serve: 6

Ingredients:

- 2 avocadoes
- 1 tsp vanilla
- 1 cup almond milk
- 1 tsp liquid stevia
- 1/2 cup unsweetened cocoa powder

Instructions:

1. In the blender, add all the listed ingredients and blend smoothly.

2. Pour blended mixture into the Popsicle molds and place in the freezer until set.

Nutrition: Calories: 130 Fat: 12 g Carbs: 7 g Sugar: 1 g Protein: 3 g Cholesterol: 0 mg

Chocolate Popsicle

Prep Time: 20 minutes

Cook Time: 10 minutes

Serve: 6

Ingredients:

- 4 oz unsweetened chocolate, chopped
- 6 drops liquid stevia
- 1 1/2 cups heavy cream

Instructions:

1. Add heavy cream into the microwave-safe bowl and microwave until it just begins the boiling.

2. Add chocolate into the heavy cream and set aside for 5 minutes.

3. Add liquid stevia into the heavy cream mixture and stir until chocolate is melted.

4. Pour mixture into the Popsicle molds and place in freezer for 4 hours or until set.

Nutrition: Calories: 198 Fat: 21 g Carbs: 6 g Sugar: 0.2 g Protein: 3 g Cholesterol: 41 mg

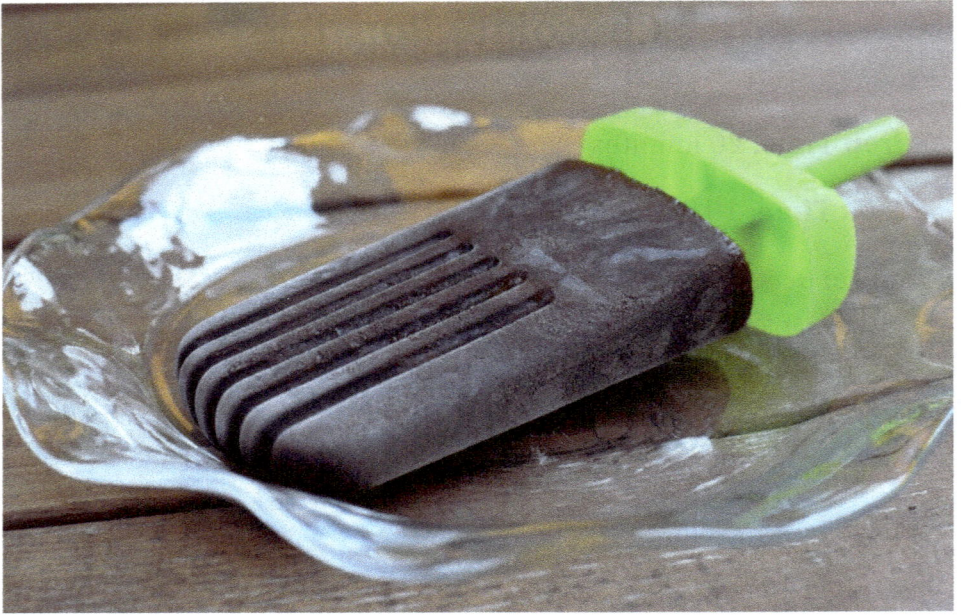

Raspberry Ice Cream

Prep Time: 10 minutes

Cook Time: 0 minutes

Serve: 2

Ingredients:

- 1 cup frozen raspberries
- 1/2 cup heavy cream
- 1/8 tsp stevia powder

Instructions:

1. Blend all the specified ingredients in a blender until smooth.

Nutrition: Calories: 144 Fat: 11 g Carbs: 10 g Sugar: 4 g Protein: 2 g Cholesterol: 41 mg

Chocolate Almond Butter Brownie

Prep Time: 10 minutes

Cook Time: 16 minutes

Serve: 4

Ingredients:

- 1 cup bananas, overripe
- 1/2 cup almond butter, melted
- 1 scoop protein powder
- 2 tbsp unsweetened cocoa powder

Instructions:

1. Preheat to 325 F the air fryer. Air fryer baking pan and set aside.

2. Preheat to 325 F the air fryer.

3. In the prepared pan, pour the batter, put it in the air fryer's basket, and cook for 16 minutes.

Nutrition: Calories: 82 Fat: 2 g Carbs: 11 g Sugar: 5 g Protein: 7 g Cholesterol: 16 mg

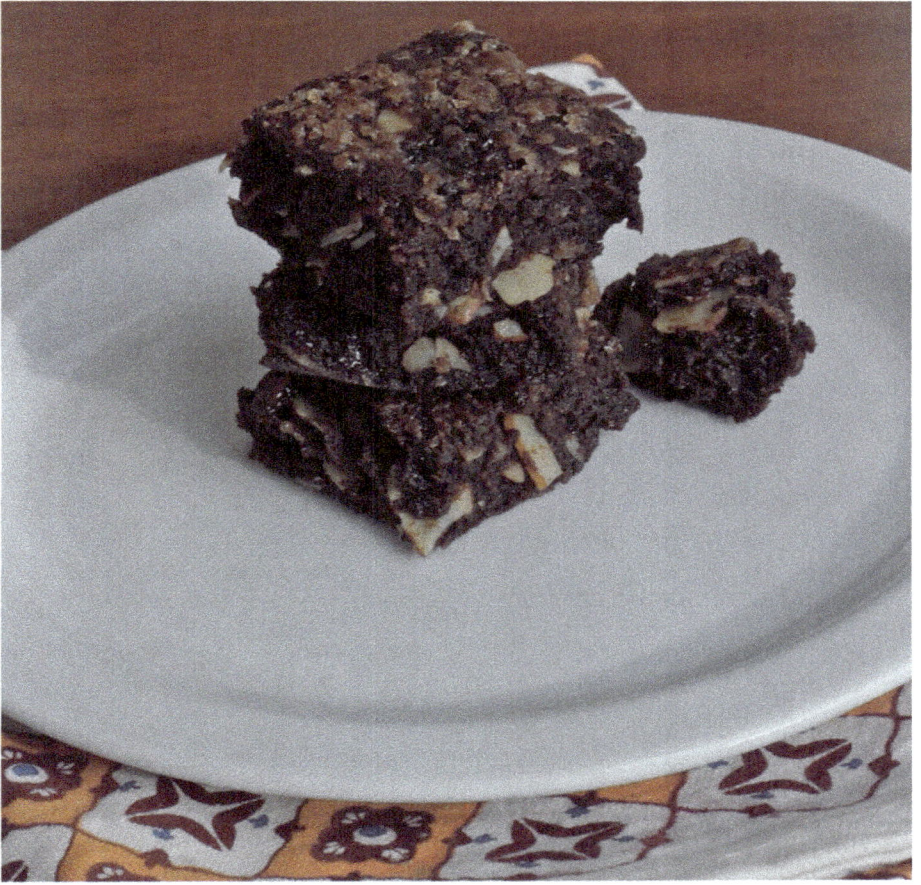

Peanut Butter Fudge

Prep Time: 10 minutes

Cook Time: 10 minutes

Serve: 20

Ingredients:

- 1/4 cup almonds, toasted and chopped
- 12 oz smooth peanut butter
- 15 drops liquid stevia
- 3 tbsp coconut oil
- 4 tbsp coconut cream
- Pinch of salt

Instructions:

1. Line baking tray with parchment paper.

2. In a pan, melt the coconut-oil over low heat. Add peanut butter, coconut cream, stevia, and salt in a saucepan. Stir well.

3. Pour fudge mixture into the prepared baking tray and sprinkle chopped almonds on top.

4. Place the tray in the refrigerator for 1 hour or until set.

Nutrition: Calories: 131 Fat: 12 g Carbs: 4 g Sugar: 2 g Protein: 5 g Cholesterol: 0 mg

Almond Butter Fudge

Prep Time: 10 minutes

Cook Time: 10 minutes

Serve: 18

Ingredients:

- 3/4 cup creamy almond butter
- 1 1/2 cups unsweetened chocolate chips

Instructions:

1. Line 8*4-inch pan with parchment paper and set aside.

2. Add chocolate chips and almond butter into the double boiler and cook over medium heat until the chocolate-butter mixture is melted. Stir well.

3. place the mixture into the prepared pan and place it in the freezer until set.

Nutrition: Calories: 197 Fat: 16 g Carbs: 7 g Sugar: 1 g Protein: 4 g Cholesterol: 0 mg

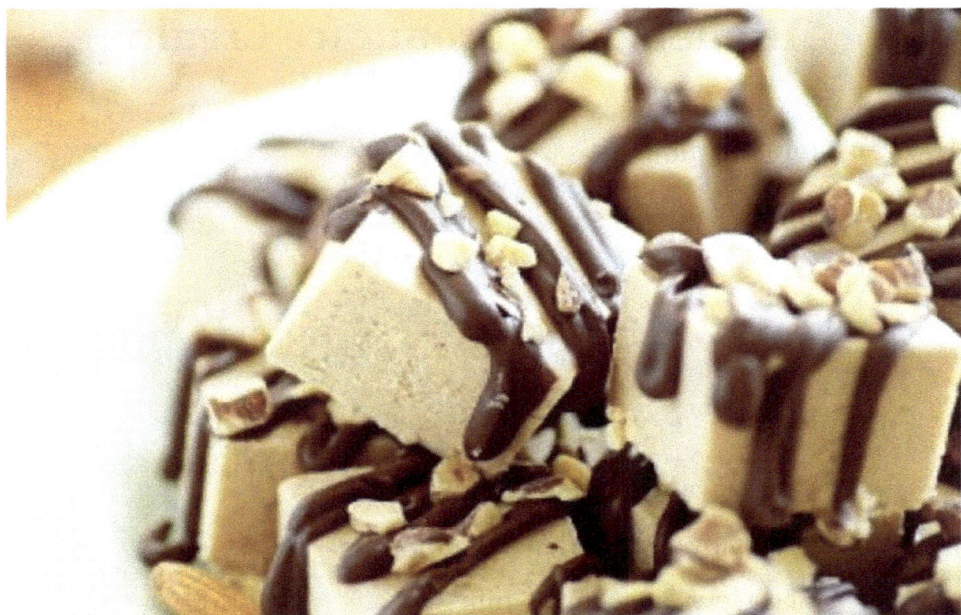

Homemade Coconut Ice Cream

Prep Time: 10 minutes

Cook Time: 95 minutes

Serve: 4

Ingredients:

- 2 cups evaporated low-fat milk
- ⅓ cup low-fat condensed milk
- 1 cup low-fat coconut milk
- 1 cup stevia/xylitol/bacon syrup
- 2 scoops whey protein concentrate
- 2 tsp. sugar-free coconut extract
- 1 tsp. dried coconut

Instructions:

1. Mix all the ingredients together in a bowl.

2. Heat the mixture over medium heat until it starts to bubble.

3. Remove from the heat and then leave the mixture to cool.

4. Chill mixture for about an hour, then freeze in ice cream maker as outlined by the manufacturer's directions.

Nutrition: Calories: 182, Fat: 2 g, Carbohydrates: 20 g, Protein: 22 g

Coconut Panna Cotta

Prep Time: 5 minutes

Cook Time: 20 minutes

Serve: 2

Ingredients:

- 2 cups skimmed milk
- 1/2 cup water
- 1 tsp. sugar-free coconut extract
- 1 envelope powdered grass-fed – organic gelatin – sugar-free
- 2 scoops whey protein isolate
- 4 tbsp. stevia/xylitol/yacon syrup
- ⅓ cup fresh raspberries
- 2 tbsp. fresh mint

Instructions:

1. In a non-stick pan, pour the milk, stevia, water, and coconut Extract.

2. Bring to a boil.

3. Slowly add the gelatin and stir well until the mixtures start to thicken.

4. When ready, divide the mix among the small silicon cups.

5. Refrigerate overnight to relax and hang up.

6. Remove through the fridge and thoroughly turn each cup over ahead of a serving plate.

7. Garnish with raspberries and fresh mint, serve and revel in.

Nutrition: Calories: 130, Fat: 3 g, Carbohydrates: 14 g, Protein: 29 g

Blueberry Lemon Cake

Prep Time: 10 minutes

Cook Time: 40 minutes

Serve: 4

Ingredients:

For the cake:

- 2/3 cup almond flour
- 5 eggs
- ⅓ cup almond milk, unsweetened
- ¼ cup erythritol
- 2 tsp. vanilla extract
- Juice of 2 lemons
- 1 tsp. lemon zest
- ½ tsp. baking soda
- Pinch of salt
- ½ cup fresh blueberries
- 2 tbsp. butter, melted

For the frosting:

- ½ cup heavy cream
- Juice of 1 lemon

- 1/8 cup erythritol

Instructions:

1. Preheat the oven to 35°F

2. In a bowl, add the almond flour, eggs, and almond milk and mix well until smooth.

3. Add the erythritol, a pinch of salt, baking soda, lemon zest, lemon juice, and vanilla extract. Mix and combine well.

4. Fold in the blueberries.

5. Use the butter to grease the pans.

6. Pour the batter into the greased pans.

7. Put on a baking sheet for even baking.

8. Put in the oven to bake until cooked through in the middle and slightly brown on the top, about 35 to 40 minutes.

9. Let cool before removing from the pan.

10. Mix the erythritol, lemon juice, and heavy cream. Mix well.

11. Pour frosting on top.

Nutrition: Calories:274, Fat: 23 g, Carbohydrates: 8 g, Protein: 9 g

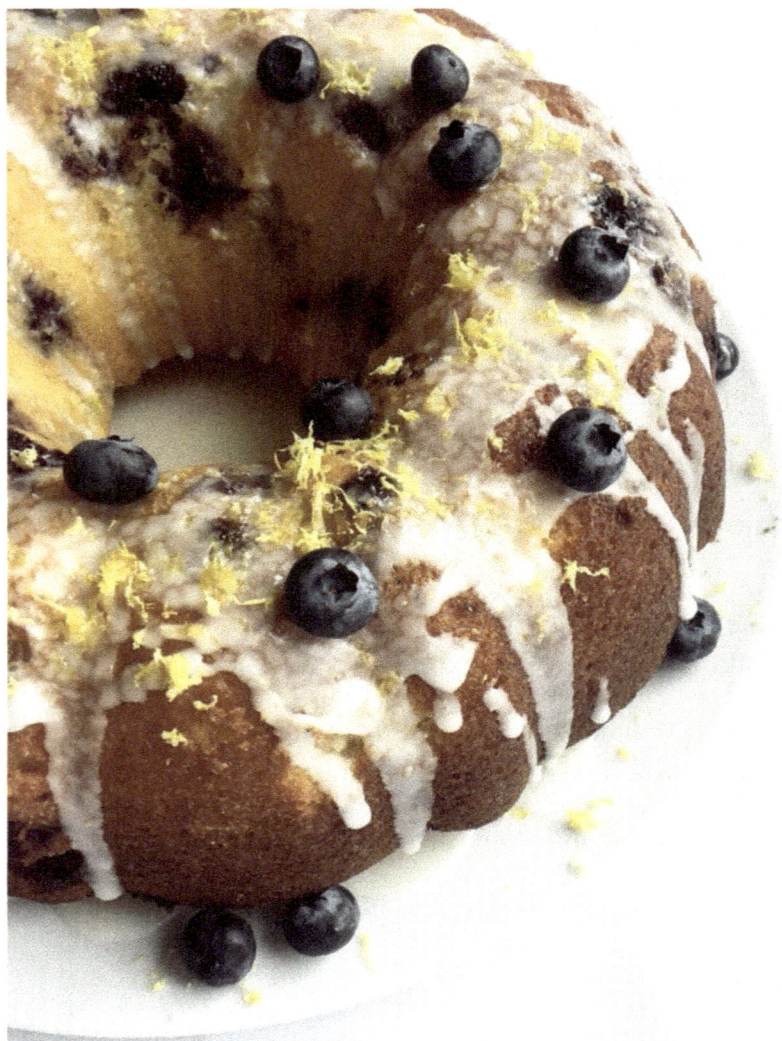

Rich Chocolate Mousse

Prep Time: 10 minutes

Cook Time: 15 minutes

Serve: 3

Ingredients:

- ¼ cup low-fat coconut cream
- 2 cups fat-free Greek-style yogurt, strained
- 4 tsp. powered cocoa, no added sugar
- 2 tbsp. stevia/xylitol/bacon syrup
- 1 tsp. natural vanilla extract

Instructions:

1. Combine all the ingredientsin a medium bowl and mix well.

2. Put individual serving bowls or glasses and refrigerate.

Nutrition: Calories: 269, Fat: 3 g, Carbohydrates: 20 g, Protein: 43 g

Raspberry Cheesecake

Prep Time: 10 minutes

Cook Time: 25 minutes

Serve: 6

Ingredients:

- 2/3 cup coconut oil, melted
- ½ cup cream cheese
- 6 eggs
- 3 tbsp. granulated sweetener
- 1 tsp. vanilla extract
- ½ tsp. baking powder
- ¾ cup raspberries

Instructions:

1. In a bowl, beat together the coconut oil and cream cheese until smooth.

2. Beat in eggs, then beat in the sweetener, vanilla, and baking powder until smooth.

3. Pour the batter into a pan and finally smooth the top. Scatter the raspberries on top.

4. Bake for 25/30 minutes or until the center is firm.

Nutrition: Calories: 176, Fat: 18 g, Carbohydrates: 3 g, Protein: 6 g

Peanut Butter Brownie Ice Cream Sandwiches

Prep Time: 2 minutes

Cook Time: 2 minutes

Serve: 2

Ingredients:

- 1 packet Medifast Brownie Mix
- 3 tablespoons water
- 1 Peanut Butter Crunch Bar or any bar of your choice
- 2 tablespoons Peanut Butter Powder
- 1 tablespoon water
- 2 tablespoons cool whip

Instructions:

1. Melt the Brownie Mix with water.

2. Add in the Peanut Butter Crunch until a dough is formed.

3. Spoon 4 dough balls on a plate and flatten using the palm of your hands.

4. Make sure that the dough is 1/4 inch thick.

5. Place in a microwave oven and cook for 2 minutes.

6. Meanwhile, mix the Peanut Butter Powder and water to form a paste.

7. Add cool whip. Leave to cool in the fridge for minimun 1 hour.

8. Take the cookies out from the microwave oven and allow it to cool.

9. Once cooled, spoon the peanut butter ice cream in between two cookies.

Nutrition: Calories per serving: 410 Cal, Protein: 8.3 g, Carbohydrates: 57.6 g, Fat: 13.2 g, Sugar: 5.3g

Chocolate Frosty

Prep Time: 20 minutes

Cook Time: 0 minutes

Serve: 4

Ingredients:

- 2 tbsp unsweetened cocoa powder
- 1 cup heavy whipping cream
- 1 tbsp almond butter
- 5 drops liquid stevia
- 1 tsp vanilla

Instructions:

1. Add cream into the medium bowl and beat using the hand mixer for 5 minutes.

2. Add remaining ingredients and blend until thick cream forms.

3. Pour in serving bowls and place them in the freezer for 30 minutes.

Nutrition: Calories: 137 Fat: 13 g Carbs: 3 g Sugar: 0.5 g Protein: 2 g, Cholesterol: 41 mg

Tiramisu Milkshake

Cook Time: 5 minutes

Serve: 1

Ingredients:

- 1 sachet Frosty Coffee Soft Serve Treat ½ cup ice
- 6 ounces plain low-fat Greek yogurt
- ½ cup almond milk
- 2 tablespoons sugar-free chocolate
- 2 tablespoons whipped topping

Instructions:

1.Place all ingredients, except the whipped, in a blender.

2.Pulse until smooth.

3.Pour in glass and top with whipped topping.

Nutrition: Calories per serving: 239; Protein: 23.7g; Carbs: 64.2g; Fat: 22.8g Sugar: 15.2g

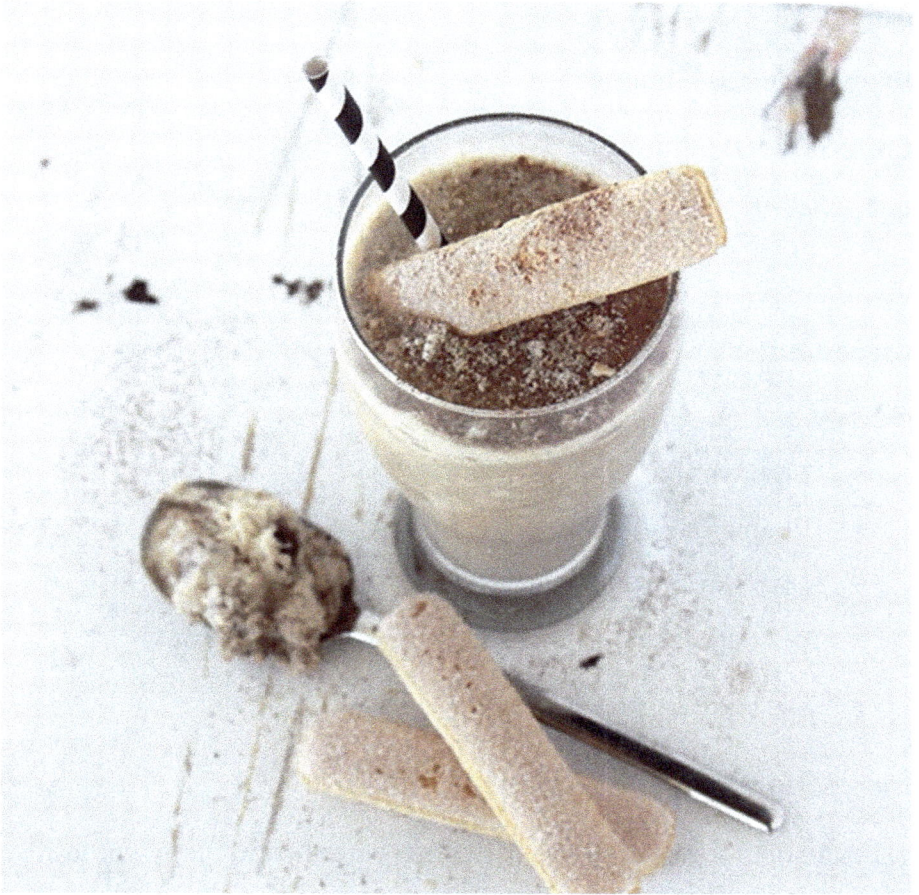

Vanilla Popsicles

Prep Time: 20 minutes

Cook Time: 0 minutes

Serve: 6

Ingredients:

- 1 tsp vanilla
- 1 cup almond milk
- 1 tsp liquid stevia
- 1/2 cup unsweetened cocoa powder

Instructions:

1. In the blender, add all the listed ingredients and blend smoothly.

2. Pour blended mixture into the Popsicle molds and place in the freezer until set.

Nutrition: Calories: 130 Fat: 12 g Carbs: 7 g Sugar: 1 g Protein: 3 g Cholesterol: 0 mg

www.ingramcontent.com/pod-product-compliance
Lightning Source LLC
Chambersburg PA
CBHW062119040426
42336CB00041B/1981